## PRESENTED TO

## FROM

## DATE

With special thanks:

To my wonderful prayer partners, Dr. Renata W. Hannah, Ph.D., and The Glory of God (Elohim's) Global Ministries, Inc. for many hours invested and so much prayer. Thank you for your faithfulness.

To my spiritual parents the late Pastor Randy Hall and Pastor Byanca Anyta Hall, Sword of the Lord Ministries for establishing the foundation of the most High God in my life. To God be the Glory.

To Bishop Donald E. Battle & Gwen Battle and Divine Faith Ministries International (DFMI).

To my daughter, Kyani and son in love Josh along with my grandkids Leighla, Kayleigh, Joshua and Liam and my son Jeremiah for filling my life with joy and giving me so much to pray about.

To Grandmother Hattie, thank you for sharing how herbs heal the body. To my mother, Sonja Mpouli for showing me how to endure.

To Denard and lovely wife Aletha, thank you for your inspiration. To Necha, for pushing me to follow my dreams.

To Zeta Hall, Jacquelyn Smith and Jonathan Hall for encouragement and always having an ear to listen to me. Thank you Aquino & India, Angela Flagg, Janella Ojeda and Calandra Anderson for being there. Many thanks to family and friends. May God Bless you all.

# DIVINE VIRTUE HEALING PLAN

## SPIRITUAL FOUNDATIONS FOR HEALTH

CHIQUILLA SCOTT, N.D.

# DIVINE VIRTUE
# HEALING PLAN

## SPIRITUAL FOUNDATIONS FOR HEALTH

# PREFACE

My perspective is that spiritual foundations for health are directly related to the study of naturopathy.  God's plan or the laws of nature are nutrition, daily exercise, plenty of sunlight, temperance, rest and Godly trust.  Naturopaths do not use drugs or surgery to heal the body.  Naturopaths believe in the prevention of sicknesses and illnesses through proper nutrition, rest, mental stability, natural stimulation and being toxin free.  These all integrate in the wholeness of man.

# TABLE OF CONTENTS

# INTRODUCTION



Spiritual foundations for health are important because it is my belief if one alters from God's plan, then the unity or harmony of the laws of life are broken. Diseases and sicknesses may be invited into the body by disregard of God's plan. I will show how naturopathy relates to biblical or scriptural foundations for health. I will research the topic through various books, articles, discussions, magazines, and (bible) The Word of God. The Word of God provides insight, maintenance and principles for the body, mind, and soul.

Jesus Christ the Healer

The scriptural principles and foundations are built upon Jesus Christ the Healer. God the Father, God the Son and the Holy Ghost. These three entities are one source. The son of God is Jesus. Jesus purpose on the earth was to save people from their sins. Jesus Christ birth centers on a virgin birth by the Holy Ghost.  His birth was fulfilled by the prophet saying,

"Therefore the Lord himself shall give you a sign; Behold, a virgin shall conceive, and bear a son, and shall call his name Immanuel" (Isaiah 7:14).

Jesus Christ is our healer and Savior.  A part of Jesus' ministry on earth; was to bring the people into unity with God the Father.  To be in unity with God; sin could not be present.  Sin is anything that separated one from the love of God.  Jesus himself took our infirmities and bare our sicknesses (Matthew 8:17).  Jesus as Christ brought tidings of salvation.  "How beautiful upon the mountains are the feet of him that bringeth good tidings, that publisheth peace, that bringeth good tidings of good, that publisheth salvation; that saith unto Zion, Thy God reigneth" (Isaiah 52:7).

The bible consists of stories of Jesus touching people and they were healed.  Jesus would speak the scriptures in the bible to the people so they would receive the gospel.  He would use opportunities of healing to testify to the truth of God's word.  Jesus suffered, died, and was buried so that we may have healing, forgiveness, and eternal life through God the Father.  "Who his own self bare our sins in his own body on a tree that we, being dead to sins, should live unto righteousness: by whose stripes ye were healed" (1Peter 2:24).

God's principles in the bible are a roadmap to give directions on how to operate the human body. The scriptures given are instructions for daily living and provide wisdom for a long life. God wants us to obey the laws and commandments to promote health. "My son, forget not my law; but let thine heart keep my commandments: for length of days, and long life, and peace, shall they add to thee" (Proverbs 3:1-2). God desires for us to fellowship with Him through prayer, reading The Word of God, singing, and praising HIM. This causes us to live in harmony with God and promotes health in the body.

The Word of God teaches us that the commandments, statutes, and judgments, which the LORD your God commanded to teach you, that ye might do them in the land whither ye go to possess it (Deuteronomy 6:1). When God's law is followed and obeyed; health is sustained. His word says, "For length of days, and long life, and peace, shall they add to thee" (Proverbs 3:2).

We are a triune being. We are created in God's image. "For there are three that bear record in heaven: the Father, the Word, and the

Holy Ghost: and these three are one" (1 John 5:7). When we accept Jesus Christ as our Lord and Savior then we become Christians. The Holy Spirit lives in the body when we become Christians. The spirit is a part of the mind of God. The Holy Spirit reveals to us God's guidance and wisdom. "What? Know ye not that your body is the temple of the Holy Ghost, which is in you, which ye have of God, and ye are not your own? For ye are bought with a price: therefore, glorify God in our body, and in your spirit, which are God's" (1 Corinthians 6:19-20).

God wants us to take good care of our body. We glorify God by taking care of our body. God desires for the body to be healed and whole. When we have true joy, peace, and knowledge of God; we want to honor Him with our whole being. Wrong habits of eating, working, breathing, resting and thinking are the basic foundation of sicknesses. "I beseech you therefore, brethren, by the mercies of God, that ye present your bodies a living sacrifice, holy, acceptable unto God, which is your reasonable service" (Romans 12:1).

# DIVINE VIRTUE HEALING PLAN

## BODY/NUTRITION

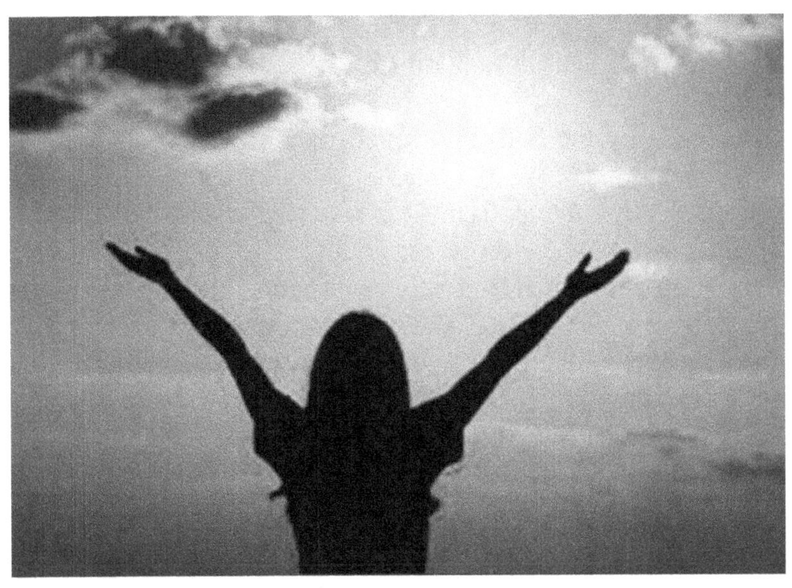

# BODY/NUTRITION

In order for the body to function and have energy it must be supplied with a food source.  You are what you eat.  A body full of nutrition or a body full of deficiencies.  The body is built like a machine and needs fuel to run.  The fuel comes from the food that we eat.

Food should provide strength, endurance and should be easily digestible.  Food provides the nutrients to the body to perform daily functions.  "Individual nutrients differ in form and function and in the amount needed by the body; however, they are all vital to our health.  The actions that involve nutrients take place on microscopic levels, and the specific processes differ greatly.  Nutrients are involved in all body processes, from combating infection to repairing tissue to thinking.  Although nutrients have different specific functions, their common functions are to keep us going" (Balch, 2010).

There are scriptural principles that relate to nutrition that God has intended to preserve health.  The four food groups contained in the

Word of God are: fruits, nuts, grains, and vegetables.  And God said, Behold, I have given you every herb bearing seed, which is upon the face of all the earth, and every tree, in the which is the fruit of a tree yielding seed; to you it shall be for meat (Genesis 1:29).

And the LORD God commanded the man, saying, Of every tree of the garden thou mayest freely eat (Genesis 2:16).

Thorns also and thistles shall it bring forth to thee; and thou shalt eat the herb of the field (Genesis 3:18).

God chose a diet of grains, fruits, nuts, and vegetables that are nourishing and healthy.

The Word of God mentioned unclean meat that was not safe to eat.  These animals were considered forbidden and unclean.  And every beast that parteth the hoof, and cleaveth the cleft into two claws, and cheweth the cud among the beasts, that ye shall eat.  Nevertheless, these ye shall not eat of them that chew cud, or of them that divide the cloven hoof; as the camel, and the hare, and the coney: for they chew the cud, but divide not the hoof; therefore, they are unclean unto you (Deuteronomy 14:6-7).  Swine is another animal that was unfit to eat because it was a scavenger.  "And the swine, though the divide the hoof, and be clovenfooted, yet he cheweth not the cud; he is unclean to you.  Of their flesh shall ye not eat, and their carcase shall ye not touch; they are unclean to you (Leviticus 11:7).  During this day and time, animal flesh could be contaminated with hormones and antibiotics.  Once the meat is consumed; it leaves toxic residue in the body's tissue which makes digestion and process of metabolism difficult.  The animal flesh could also be diseased and bring about disease, cancer and toxin to the person consuming.  Consuming high animal protein produces premature aging and short life expectancy. "We should be aware of those who wish to persuade us that our diet can be adequate and satisfying when it consists of processed, preserved, dead, embalmed and otherwise devitalized foods, despite the fact that their preparation or consumption might be more convenient at times" (Ballentine, 2007).  The food that affects the body also affects the mind and the soul.

Food can be stimulants or narcotics.  Stimulants and narcotics can be harmful to the body, irritate the stomach, excite the nerves, and poison the blood.  Some examples are tea and coffee, condiments, tobacco, and alcoholic beverages.  Tea and coffee causes the nervous system to overreact.   Condiments are food items like spices, mustards, and pepper.  Condiments are irritants that affect the nervous system. Tobacco excites, paralyzes the nerves and overall poisonous to the body.  Alcoholic beverages can induce drunkenness.  The Word of God speaks against being drunk with wine.  Do not drink wine nor strong drink, thou, nor thy sons with thee, when ye go into the tabernacle of the congregation, lest ye die it shall be a statute forever throughout your generations (Leviticus 10:9).  The overreaction excites the brain and continued use of stimulants and narcotics results in headaches, indigestion, and heart issues.

Today, people eat to satisfy the taste buds or palate on the tongue.  These foods have little to no nutritional value and causes toxins to form in the body.  Proper nutrition is not received because the food is processed or cooked.  The body will break down and malfunction if there is a deficiency of nutrients.  God's principles are designed for the body to self heal, to be healthy and well balanced.  In order for the body, organs, cells, and tissue to function properly; one must have a healthy and nutritious diet.  "Those who have rejected God's principles of healthful living tend to cite isolated examples of "abuse" or over-emphasis" of using natural foods as proof that the entire practice is off balance.  Many such critics subscribe to the notion that people should leave health matters entirely to medical doctors, maintaining that reliance on medications and prescriptions is more "normal" than trying to protect or maintain one's own health by natural means.  In order to protect their own weak position, thy ridicule others as health fanatics" (Cobb, 2002).

# NOTES

# DIVINE VIRTUE HEALING PLAN

## BODY/EXERCISE

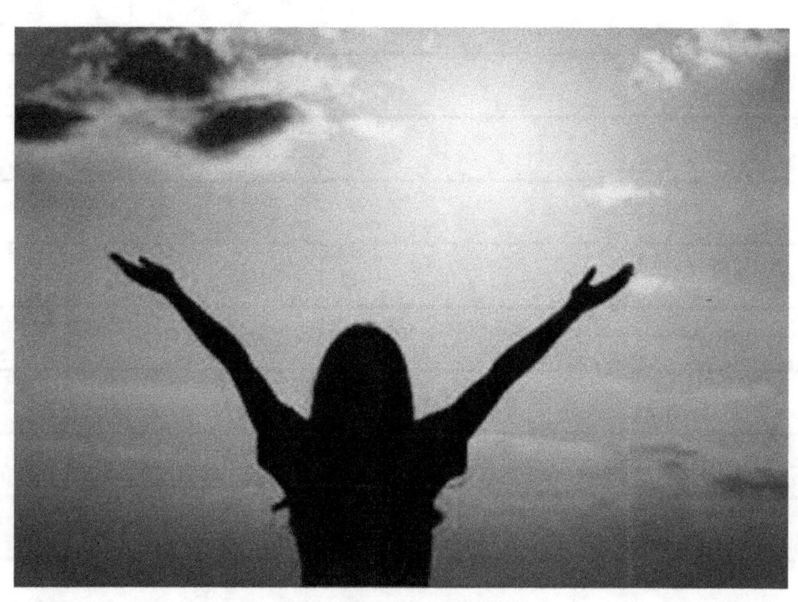

# BODY/EXERCISE

Exercise as it relates to the body is physical movement. Exercise helps to improve and preserve health.  The body was created to function and to do work.  The body depends on development and strength through exercises.  In the sweat of thy face shalt thou eat bread till thou return unto the ground; for out of it wast thou taken for dust thou art and unto dust shalt thou return (Genesis 3:19).  And the LORD God took the man and put him into the Garden of Eden to dress it and to keep it (Genesis 2:15).  God created the man to work or exercise to cause the body to release toxins.

Exercising causes the blood to circulate throughout the body and helps to eliminate the blood of toxins.  It increases vitality which is necessary to health.  When exercise is performed in pure fresh air, it gives the lungs oxygen which is necessary for life and health.  Exercise causes the body to build muscle mass.  "Muscles compromise approximately 50% of body weight" (Takahashi, 1989).   Physical activity on a consistent basis will improve muscle strength and boost endurance.

People that are inactive have poor circulation which can elevate the blood pressure.  Society, technology, computers, television, and social media have influenced people to become inactive which is detrimental for the body.  Although most people are inactive; they can get exercise from working in the garden, household duties and at their workplace environment.  An inactive body does not have blood that circulates freely.  If the body is inactive, it will not rid the body of toxins, then diseases and illnesses will take over.

"Most of the medical symptoms caused by inactivity are well known and they are alarming.  A body that isn't used deteriorates.  The lungs become inefficient, the heart grows weaker, the blood vessels less pliable, the muscles lose tone, and the body generally weakens throughout, leaving it vulnerable for a whole catalog of illnesses and disease.  Your whole system for delivering oxygen almost literally shrivels up" (Gods principle of healthful living).

It is important to incorporate aerobic exercises such as walking, running, swimming, and cycling as part as a daily regimen. These exercises revitalize the body and yield great benefits. They will also condition the lungs and the heart to distribute oxygen to the body. The body is dependent on the air that we breathe. Aerobic exercise rejuvenates the cardiovascular system.

# NOTES

# DIVINE VIRTUE HEALING PLAN

## BODY/SUNLIGHT

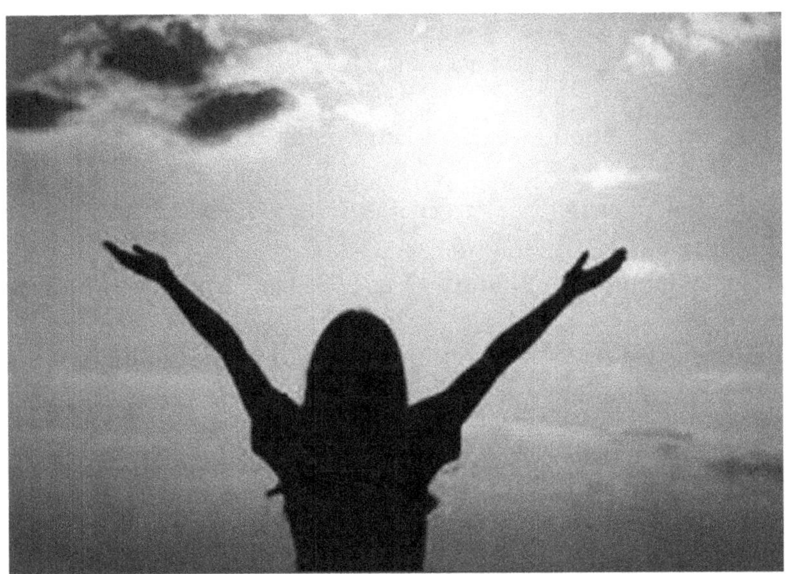

# BODY/SUNLIGHT

The scriptural principle for the sun is that it is a healing agent. The sun is a natural health remedy. The Bible states that, "But unto you that fear my name shall the Sun of righteousness arise with healing in his wings; and ye shall go forth, and grow up as calves of the stall" (Malachi 4:2).

Sunlight has an impact upon the body. The sunlight causes a person to perspire and sweat. When one sweats or perspires, it brings out toxins and germs that are in the body. The sun is important in producing vitamin D. Vitamin D is produced when one is in the sun and the sun is absorbed through the skin. Vitamin D function is to aid in calcium absorption in the diet. Calcium is important in forming bones and teeth. When there is a lack of vitamin D then rickets can develop lack of sleep and diarrhea.

It has been researched that over exposure to sunlight causes cancer. If one is constantly in the sun, then it will burn the skin.

Exposure to increased sunlight will produce excess vitamin D. Skin cancer is formed in the absence of vitamin F. Vitamin F is taking into the body through fats and oils in the diet. The combination of a diet high in fat and excessive sun exposure can cause skin cancer. Vitamin F regenerates the skin. Before sun exposure, protect the skin with sunscreen lotion and limit the time in direct sunlight to thirty minutes.

## NOTES

# DIVINE VIRTUE
# HEALING PLAN

## BODY/TEMPERANCE

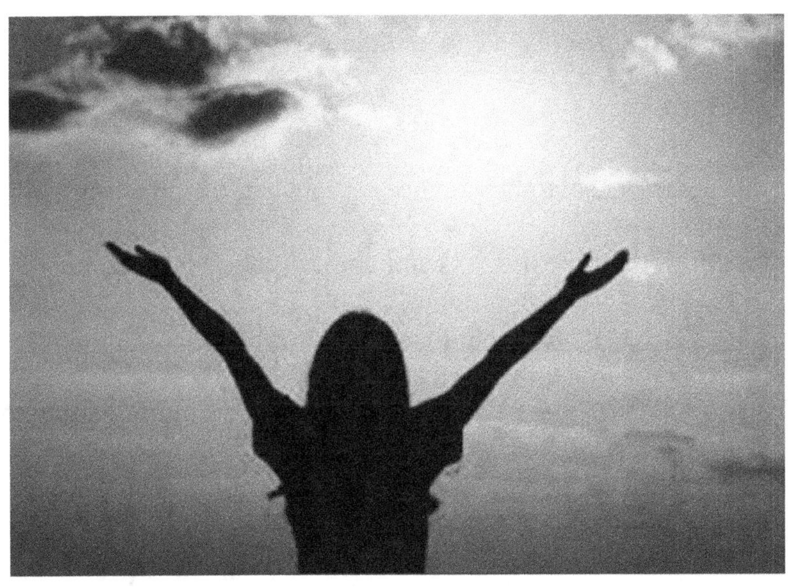

# BODY/TEMPERANCE

The scriptural principle as it relates to temperance is self-control.  Health can be preserved through self-control.  But the fruit of the Spirit is love, joy, peace, longsuffering, gentleness, goodness, faith, meekness, temperance: against such there is no law (Galatians 5:22-23).  God wants us to exercise self-control in every area of life.  And to knowledge temperance; and to temperance patience; and to patience godliness (2 Peter 1:6).

We should have temperance or self-control in eating, working, and anything that we do.  Temperance can be divided into two principles.  The first principle of temperance abstains completely from things that are harmful and bad.  The second principle of temperance is to use moderation in things that are good for you.

# NOTES

# DIVINE VIRTUE HEALING PLAN

## BODY/REST

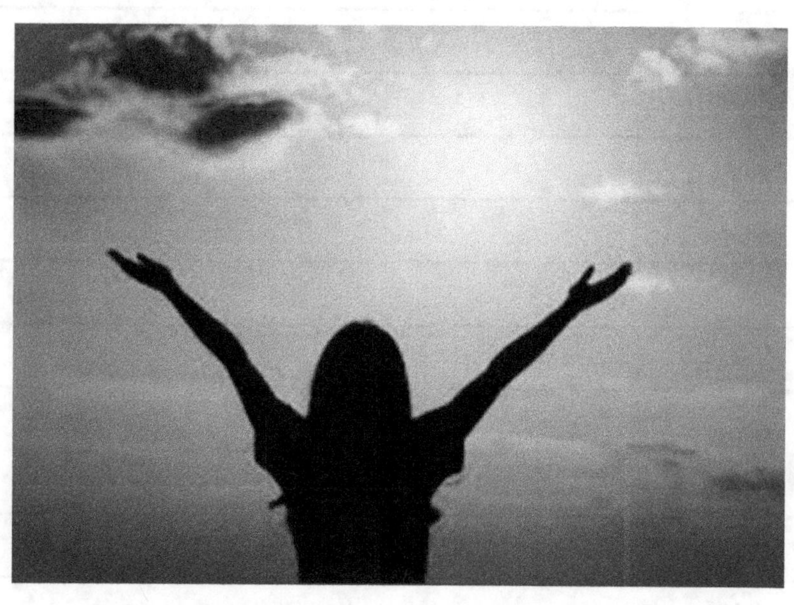

# BODY/REST

Rest is recovery from day-to-day activities. Websters' dictionary define rest as the act or period of taking one's ease after working or being active, as by sleeping and keeping still. Rest is freedom from worry, trouble and pain. To be worry free is a peaceful mind. We live in a society where there is constant "on the go activities". One must slow down to cause the body to have rest so that the body is rejuvenated, and stress level is reduced.

There are scriptural principles surrounding rest. Come unto me, all ye that labour and are heavy laden and I will give you rest. Take my yoke upon you and learn of me; for I am meek and lowly in heart: and ye shall find rest unto your souls. For my yoke is easy, and my burden is light (Matthew 11:28-30). As one work or overwork; he would become tired and weary. It's important to stop what you are doing and rest and meditate on the goodness of the Lord.

There are three different types of rest presented in The Word of God. The three types of rest are: rest, relaxation, and worship. One form of rest is sleep. When one is asleep the body rebuilds the immune system that helps fight against germs and diseases.  I will both lay me down in peace, and sleep: for thou, LORD, only makest me dwell in safety (Psalm 4:8).  A person can become sick through overworking and not getting proper sleep or rest.  Proper sleep or rest is sleeping six to eight hours a night depending on the individual.  When thou liest down, thou shalt not be afraid: Yea, thou shall lie down, and thy sleep shall be sweet (Proverbs 3:24).  God wants us to enjoy sleep.  It is vain for you to rise up early, to sit up late, to eat the bread of sorrows: for he giveth his beloved sleep (Psalm 127:2).

Relaxation is another form of rest.  And he said unto them, Come ye yourselves apart into a desert place, and rest awhile: for there were many coming and going, and they had no leisure so much as to eat (Mark 6:31).  Leisurely relaxing means being carefree.  There remaineth therefore a rest to the people of God.  For he that is entered into his rest, he also hath ceased from his own works, as God did from his.  Let us labour therefore to enter into that rest, lest any man fall after the same example of unbelief (Hebrews 4:9-11).  Nature gives a sense of relaxation by one picking flowers, walking through the greenery, and listening to the sounds in nature.

The third principle of relaxation is worship.  The Word of God principle of worshipping God is surrendering everything to God. You can worship God by setting aside time to pray/meditate, read the bible, and singing unto God. The Word of God mentions setting aside a day to rest. During that day of rest: do not work but only worship him. But the seventh day is to the sabbath of the LORD thy God: in it thou shalt not do any work, thou, nor thy son, nor thy daughter, thy manservant, nor thy maid servant, nor thy cattle, nor thy stranger that is within thy gates (Exodus 20:10). God gives commandment to worship Him. By doing so, we follow the principle, and it is one of the ways of keeping sicknesses and diseases from entering the body. The body, mind and soul are strengthened from being in the presence of God.

# NOTES

# DIVINE VIRTUE HEALING PLAN

## BODY/TRUST IN GOD

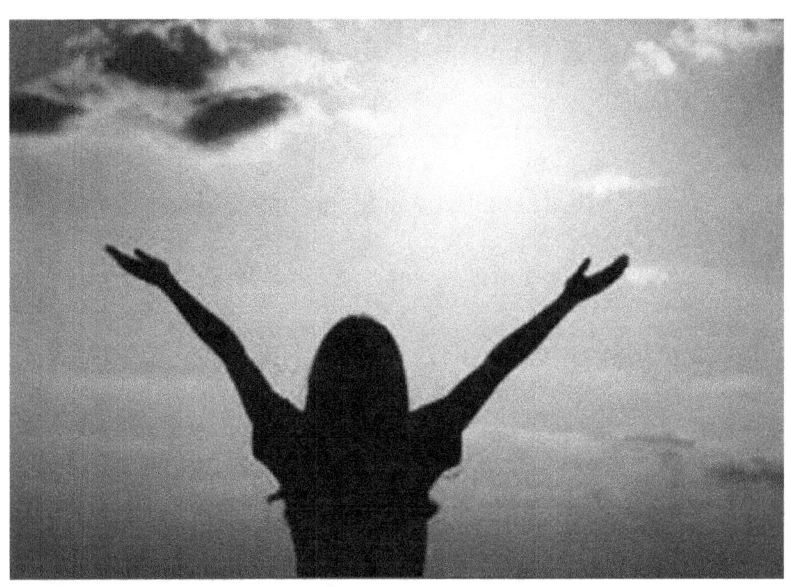

# BODY/TRUST IN GOD

God has loved us with an unconditional love. Unconditional love is not based on situations or circumstances but is everlasting not regarding particular outcomes. I believe that to mean, that God loves us no matter what. Where there is sin; sin separates us from God. God's heart of love remains open to us. When love is unconditional it brings forth a level of trust and dependency. With this love, God wants us to trust him with our entire being and our whole heart. God's love is refreshing and strengthening day by day. God has reassured us in The Word of God, Romans 8:38-39:

For I am persuaded, that neither death, nor life, nor angels, nor principalities, nor powers, nor things present, nor things to come, nor height, nor depth, nor any other creature, shall be able to separate us from the love of God, which is in Christ Jesus our Lord.

God allows the trust to build in a deep relationship with such a great show of love. Casting all your care upon him; for he careth for you (1 Peter 5:7). Trust in the LORD with all thine heart; and lean not to thine own understanding. In all thy ways acknowledge him, and he shall direct thy paths. Be not wise in thy own eyes: fear the LORD and depart from evil. It shall be health to thy navel, and marrow to thy bones (Proverbs 3:5-8). Jesus commanded us to love God with all our heart, soul, mind, and strength (Bright, 2002, pg. 19). By having a dependency on a supernatural and omnipotent being eliminates self-dependency.

An active relationship with God, through Jesus Christ, benefits physical and emotional health. A relationship with God consists of prayer, reading the bible and following his commandments and statutes. And said, If thou wilt diligently hearken to the voice of the LORD thy God, and wilt do that which is right in his sight, and wilt give ear to his commandments, and keep his statutes, I will put none of these diseases upon thee, which I have brought upon the Egyptians: for I am the Lord that healeth thee (Exodus 15:26).

Science has proven now, that people who trust in God, and have faith, come through illnesses and surgeries better than those who do not trust in God. Trusting in God gives one a sense of peace and eliminates anxiety which leads to stress. As pressure and stress bear down on me, I find joy in your commands (Psalm 119:143, New Living Translation).

Trusting in God relieves stress. When there is no trust in God, or one is self-sufficient then stress is elevated. Stress leads to worry. Meditating and reading The Word of God reduces stress. Worry weighs a person down; an encouraging word cheers a person up (Proverbs 12:25 New Living Translation).

Stress leads to high blood pressure. High blood pressure is caused by elevated heart rate, constricted blood vessels, plaque, sodium retention and toxic buildup. Stress can be regulated by trusting in God, regulating salt intake, avoiding high cholesterol foods, exercising, avoiding smoking and excessive intake of alcoholic beverages.

# NOTES

# DIVINE VIRTUE HEALING PLAN

## BODY/AIR

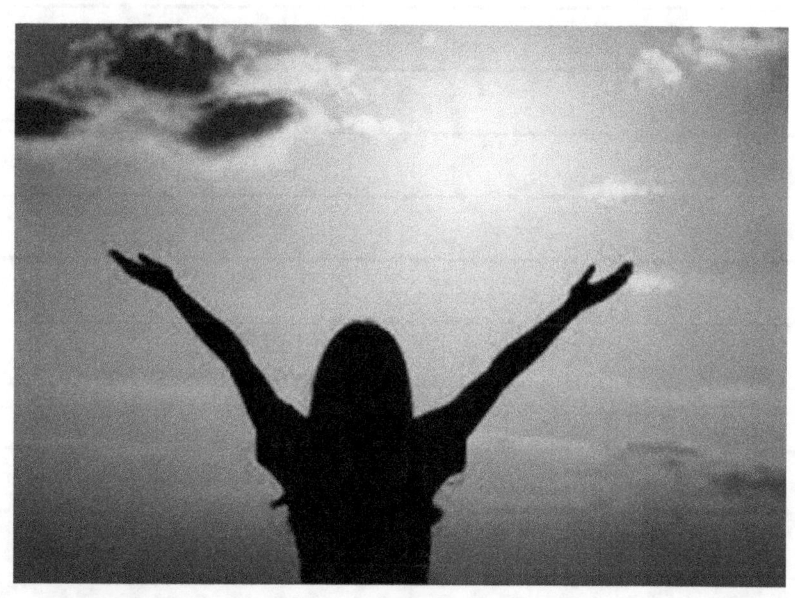

# BODY/AIR

~ ~ ~

Air is essential and is needed to survive.  Air is what we breathe.  Air is made up of oxygen and essential to life.  God has given us the breath of life.  And the Lord God formed man of the dust of the ground, and breathed into his nostrils the breath of life; and man became a living soul (Genesis 2:7).  He himself gives life and breath to everything, and he satisfies every need.  "Neither is worshipped with men's hands, as though he needed any thing, seeing he giveth to all life, and breath, and all things" (Acts 17:25).

Fresh air is needed to increase oxygen levels in the body.  It is the purifier and supporter of blood.  The blood is purified through the air.  It is important to inhale fresh air continuously day and night.  Fresh air is needed for the skin and lungs.  Air is a life supporting agent rich in oxygen.

# NOTES

# DIVINE VIRTUE HEALING PLAN

## BODY/WATER

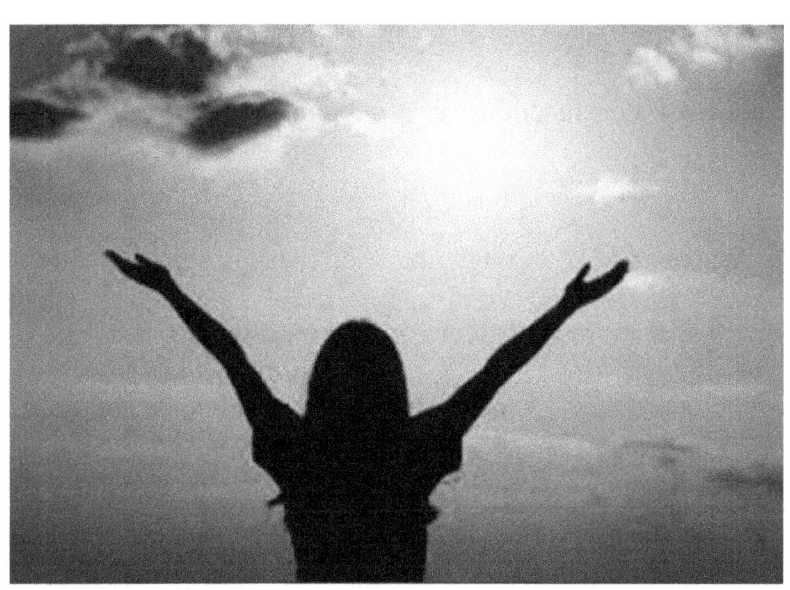

# BODY/WATER

Water is essential for life. Water is vital for normal bodily processes. However, people do not intake enough water on a daily basis. According to the American Dietetic Association, it's not eight glasses of water a day; its eight 8-ounce servings.

Many health problems are caused by toxins within the body and blood stream. Water can help flush toxins and heal the body of impurities. Water functions as a supplier, regulator, and beneficial factor.

Water supplied throughout the body helps digestion, circulation, absorption, and excretion. Water aids in carrying nutrients and oxygen throughout the body. One common health issue is kidney stones. Kidney stones can be prevented with increase water consumption. Kidney stones are formed through mineral and salts. Water dilutes urine and help prevents the concentration of the mineral salts.

Water regulates and maintains body temperature. Water is lost through sweat or perspiration. Water level must be balanced if one is very active. It is important to stay hydrated to protect the skin. One sign that the body is dehydrated through the skin is the appearance of visible wrinkles.

Water is beneficial by promoting weight loss, improves short term memory and slowing the aging process. When enough water is not consumed, the body produces a hormone called aldosterone. Aldosterone is a hormone that causes tissues to hold onto every molecule of liquid water. A decrease in water increases body fat deposits.

Water is important inside the body and outside the body. Water is needed on a daily basis to prevent dehydration. The body warns of dehydration as a sign of being thirsty. Sometimes hunger is a sign of dehydration. Water can be lost through breathing, sweating, through the skin and the kidneys.

Water is vital to the human body. Water is classified as: bottled, tap, natural spring and distilled. "Distilled water is considered the purest water, but is also divorces from all nutrients" (Lepore, 1985). A person should drink half their weight in ounces of water daily. Health professionals recommend drinking distilled water. "Once consumed, steam distilled water leaches inorganic minerals rejected by the cells and tissues out of the body" (Balch, pg. 53).

Water is important outside the body. The Word of God talks about the water in the pool of Bethesda and how it was used to purify and heal the body. For an angel went down at a certain season into the pool and troubled the water: whosoever then first after the troubling of water stepped in was made whole of whatsoever disease he had (John 5:4). It is a common practice to soak the body in a bathtub of warm water and Epsom salt. This combination relaxes the joints and muscles to reduce pain and inflammation.

# NOTES

# DIVINE VIRTUE HEALING PLAN

## MIND

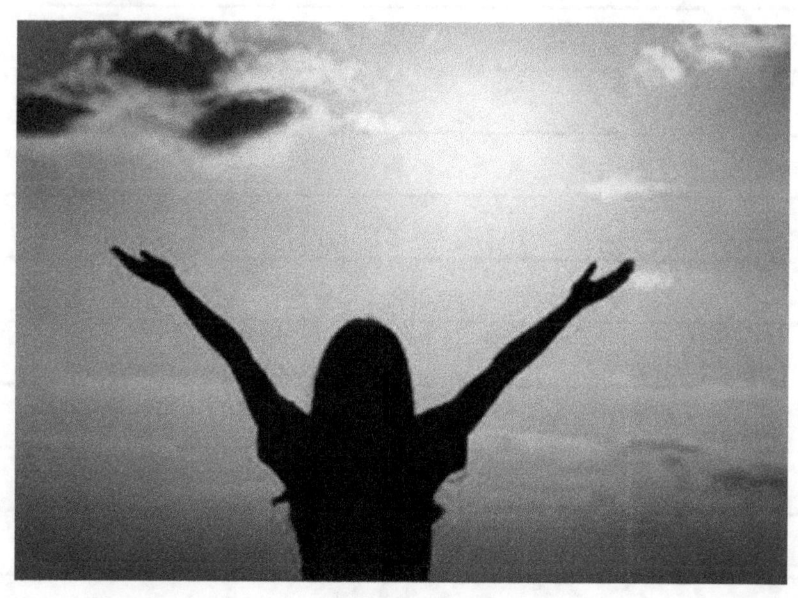

# MIND

~ 39 ~

We are a triune being: body, mind, and soul.  One of the scriptural principles of health involves the mind.  To have optimal health physically in the body begins with the mind.

The Word of God says, "Let this mind be in you, which was also in Christ Jesus" (Philippians 2:5).

Christian's scriptural foundation belief in a higher authority or supernatural source of God being the Creator.  God is the divine power. Christians believe that they are created in the image of Jesus Christ, who is the Son of God.

"For who hath known the mind of the Lord, that he may instruct him? But we have the mind of Christ" (1 Corinthians 2:16).

The mind can be free and experience happiness which produces joy and peace to the whole being.  Faith, courage, hope, and love promotes health and prolongs life.  A contented mind, a cheerful spirit is the body and strength to the soul.  "A merry heart doeth good like a medicine: but a broken spirit drieth the bone" (Proverbs 17:22).

The mind relates to the brain. The mind can consist of feelings, attitudes, thoughts, memories, beliefs, and imaginations. The brain is the overall driving force located in the body that deciphers the mind. The mind functions through the brain nerves which connect with every part of the body. The skull houses the brain. The brain consists of cerebrum, cerebellum which houses the brain stem. The brain stem holds the pituitary gland which controls the hormones. The brain stem can also be divided into the thalamus and hypothalamus. The thalamus is part of the brain that is triggered when a thought occurs; it decodes the information and channels it through the amygdala which stores memories. The amygdala alerts the body of emotional response to a thought. The amygdala holds every thought that has ever been experienced. The amygdala safeguards, reminds and protect the emotions from issues reoccurring.

Thoughts can be positive and negative. God's instructions: "Casting down imaginations, and every high thing that exalteth itself against the knowledge of God and bringing into captivity every thought to the obedience of Christ" (2 Corinthians 10:5). When negative thoughts occur; it causes the body to continuously release downer chemicals. Some negative emotions are produced from these hormones: hate, fear frustration, anger, guilt or envy. A sound heart is the life of the flesh, but envy is the rottenness of the bones. "For as he thinketh in his heart, so is he: Eat and drink, saith he to thee: but his heart is not with thee" (Proverbs 23:7). Negative emotions are toxic and cause downer chemicals to affect the brains nerve cells. The hormones produced from toxic can affect the metabolism of the cells in the body and cause difficulty in retrieving memories.

Our emotional pain can trigger physical pain or damage. Researchers have linked toxic thoughts to the heart and vascular problems, gastrointestinal problems, headaches, skin conditions, intestinal tract disorders and immune impairment. Consider this from Dr. Caroline Leaf's Who Switched off my brain?

"Research shows 87% of illnesses can be attributed to our thought life and approximately 13% to diet genetics and environment. Studies conclusively link more chronic disease (lifestyle diseases) to epidemic of toxic emotions in our culture. These toxic emotions can cause migraines, hypertension, strokes, cancers, skin problems, diabetes, infection, and allergies, just to name a few" (Wright, 2011).

Thoughts can be positive.  When a person experiences happiness, joy, excitement or peace the brain secretes hormones or chemicals making the body feel good.  The hormones help control emotions and strengthen the cells in the body.  Love, hope, faith, courage, and sympathy promote long life and health.  A contented mind and a cheerful spirit is health to the body and strengthen the soul.  Positive thoughts bring about positive feelings.  "Finally, brethren, whatsoever things are true, whatsoever things are honest, whatsoever things are just, whatsoever things are pure, whatsoever things are lovely, whatsoever things are of a good report; if there be any virtue, and if there be any praise, think on these things" (Philippians 4:8).  Having control over your thoughts, thinking positive and stimulating the mind can promote long life and health.  Controlling the thoughts that come into the mind can change character.

The brain holds the thought process in the mind.  The brain produces and secretes hormones into the body.  Positive thoughts can produce an emotion of joy and happiness.  Negative thoughts can produce toxic emotions.  God's word gives us the standard for right thoughts.  "So, what exactly are thoughts?  Well, they're the ways in which we're conscious of things.  They're made up of our memories, our perceptions, our beliefs" (Wright, 2011). "Each behavior begins this way: A thought stimulates an electrical response, which produces emotion; emotion results in an attitude; attitude produces behavior" (Wright, 2011).

You must take control of your mind. "Many of the diseases from which men suffer are the result of mental depression. Grief, anxiety, discontent, remorse, guilt, distrust, all tend to break down life forces and to invite decay and death" (White, 2007). If you do not take control of your mind, then it is subject to the devil's will. A big part of standing against the enemy of our souls is taking control over our minds.

# NOTES

# DIVINE VIRTUE HEALING PLAN

## BODY/SOUL

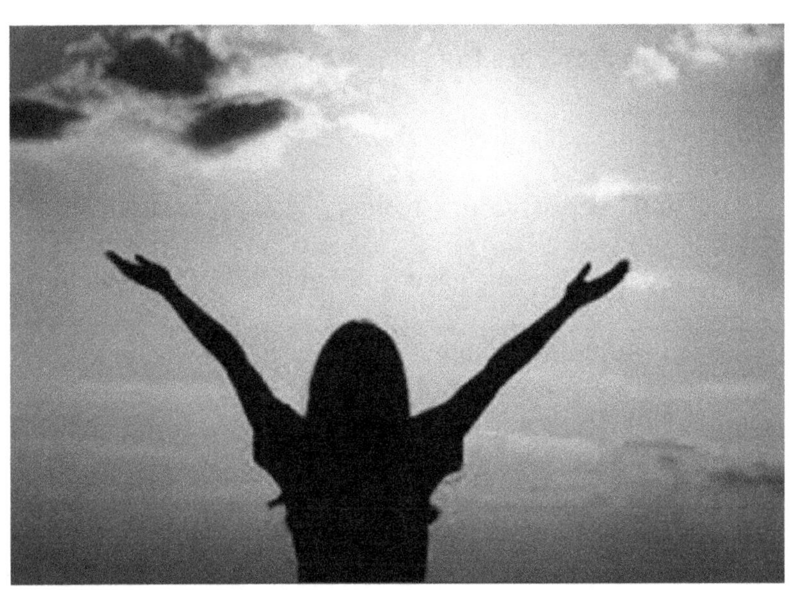

# SOUL

Christ is the restorer. "And he shall be unto thee a restorer of thy life, and a nourisher of thine old age" (Ruth 4:15). Obeying the laws of health to perfect holiness; honors God. He will impart to them His life. When we present Christ, we are imparting a power, a strength that is of value; for it comes from above. This is the true healing for the body and soul.

The soul represents our feelings, will and emotions. "When God made us in his image he gave us a mind, a will and emotions. The mind gives us the ability to think. Our emotions provide the ability to feel. Our will allows us the opportunity to choose" (Wright, 2011).

As living beings, we rely on our emotions to influence our lives. Emotions are also driven by the thought process. When we begin to align our life to GOD's word then the focus on SELF diminishes. Growing and having dependency in God will build strength, influence the mind, and fill the soul with zeal.

God wants us to have victory in our soul. "Nay, in all these things, we are more than conquerors through him that loved us" (Romans 8:37). We must yield our emotions and feelings and replace them with the law of God's word.  And if thou draw out thy soul to the hungry and satisfy the afflicted soul; then shall thy light rise in obscurity and thy darkness be as the noon day (Isaiah 58:10).

# NOTES

# DIVINE VIRTUE HEALING PLAN

## NATUROPATHY VS MEDICAL DOCTOR

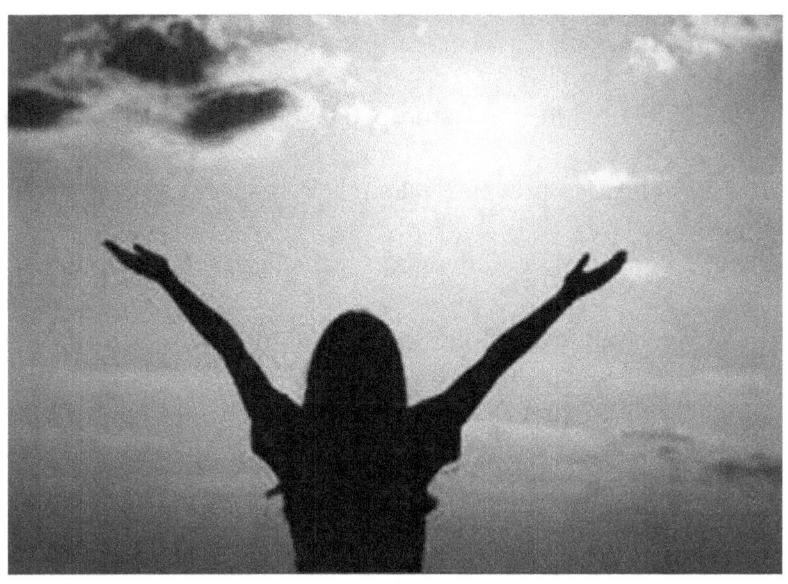

# NATUROPATHY VS MEDICAL DOCTOR

Naturopathy, to quote Benedict Lust, "is a distinct school of healing, employing the beneficent agency of Nature's forces of water, air, sunlight, earth, power, electricity, magnetism, exercise, rest, proper diet, various kinds of mechanical treatment and mental and moral science" (Thiel, 2000). Naturopaths do not practice medicine. Naturopaths believe in prevention and that the body can heal itself.

Unlike medical doctors, naturopaths believe in the prevention of diseases by teaching natural laws of living and applying it day to day. Naturopaths believe that drugs do not cure. Drugs relieve pain and change the symptoms. Naturopaths search out the cause of the disease or illness.

Medical doctors are trained to treat symptoms related to the diseases. Medical doctors study medicine and do not study foods that heal. Wrong eating and faulty diets bring about most sicknesses and diseases. Medical doctors diagnose people based on symptoms. Drugs treat the symptoms. Symptoms may change frequently; therefore, a smorgasbord of drugs may be prescribed. Drugs may appear to fix a problem but if there is no immediate relief, then another medicine is offered, and the cycle continues. Therefore, the drug does not cure but change the location and form of the disease.

The body can become immune to drugs depending on how often the drugs are being administered. The drugs presented to the body over a period of time make the body toxic and enzyme deficient. The toxicity of the poisonous drugs brings lifelong illnesses. Drugs and surgeries are only temporarily fixes and cannot heal the body.

It's important to address the problems of the body by changing habits. Wholeness and health will be restored once the cause is recognized, and habits are changed that created the problem. Overall health is sustained by removing poisons and toxics from the body. Once these are removed; then deficient enzymes will be rebuilt.

Naturopaths educate people on the principles of health of the body which includes pure air, sunlight, rest, exercise, proper diet and the use of water. Naturopaths believe in the healing power of nature. People become sick because they have violated nature's laws.

Scriptural foundations of health relate to naturopathy and God's word.

If one is obedient to the law of God's word, they will reap the reward of

health in the body, mind, and soul.

# NOTES

# DIVINE VIRTUE HEALING PLAN

**ARE NATUROPATHS' QUACKS?**

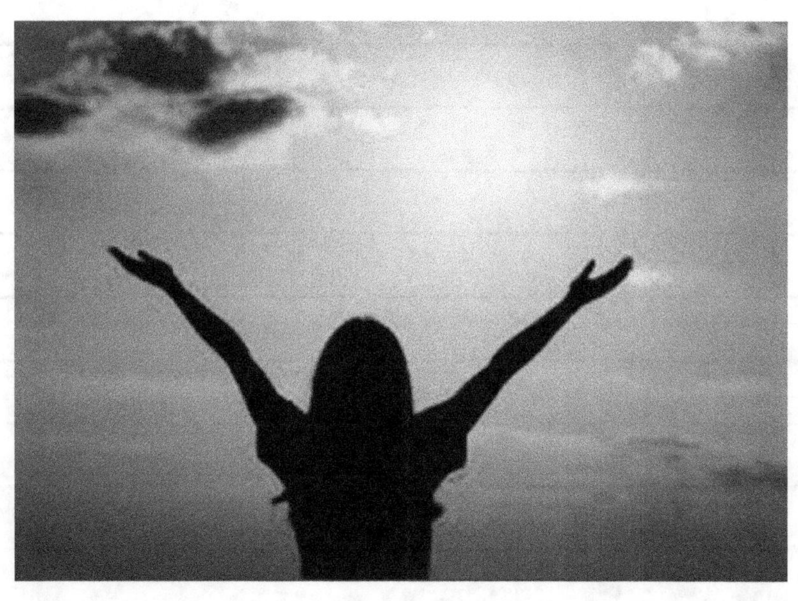

# ARE NATUROPATHS' QUACKS?

~ 55 ~

Naturopaths have been criticized for their belief in natural healing. Naturopaths have been called quacks. A quack is an untrained person practicing medicine fraudulently. In fact, naturopaths do not practice medicine at all.

"This brings us to a popular "system" of alternative medicine: naturopathy. From the headline, you know my bias here: naturopathy is not medicine or science, but more akin to religion. In Colorado and Michigan bills are under consideration to allow naturopaths to have many of the same privileges as doctors" (Lipson, 2016).

Naturopaths believe in the prevention of illnesses and diseases. Naturopaths believe that the body can heal itself. Naturopaths instruct clients by...."identifying the cause of problems, eliminating toxins, recommending substances to deal with deficiencies and stimulating the body's own natural healing abilities" (Thiel, 2000).

# NOTES

# DIVINE VIRTUE HEALING PLAN

## CONCLUSION

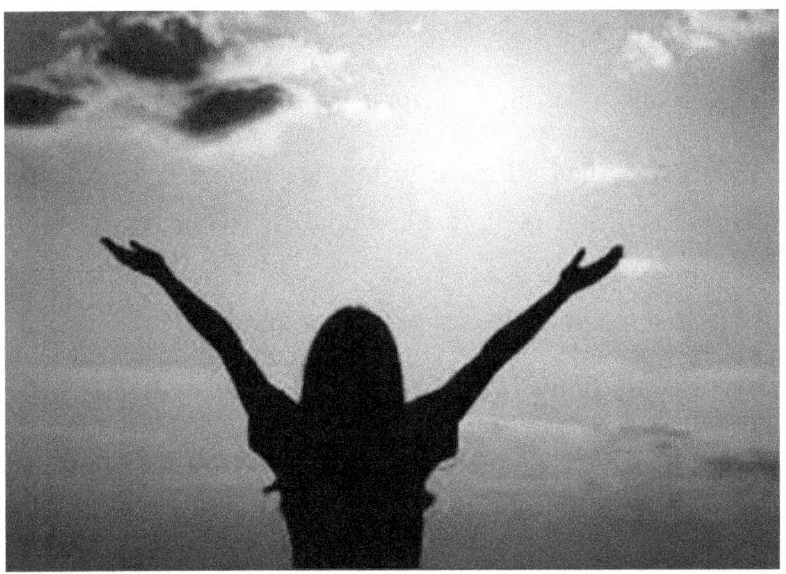

# CONCLUSION

Scriptural foundations for health are related to naturopathy. The laws of God correlate to the belief behind naturopathy. The laws of God regulate the body. When the laws of God are broken and violated then diseases and sicknesses result. Naturopathy uses fresh air, pure water, sunlight, and proper food supply to cure diseases without the use of drugs, poisons, or toxins.

Health is a foundation built not only on food and exercise. Health also consists of other factors: relationship with God, rest, and mental clarity. When all these factors are balanced then it promotes living healthy.

Understanding scriptural principles and applying them to day to day living integrates the wholeness of man as it relates to naturopathy. Naturopathy healing sources are made up of the healing agencies as air, sunshine, water, heat, electricity, manipulations, rest, natural vital foods, organic vitamins, organic minerals in conjunction with cleansing and eliminating processes of other physical and mental cultures (Thiel, 2000).

# NOTES

# NOTES

# DIVINE VIRTUE HEALING PLAN

## MEDITATE AND REFLECT

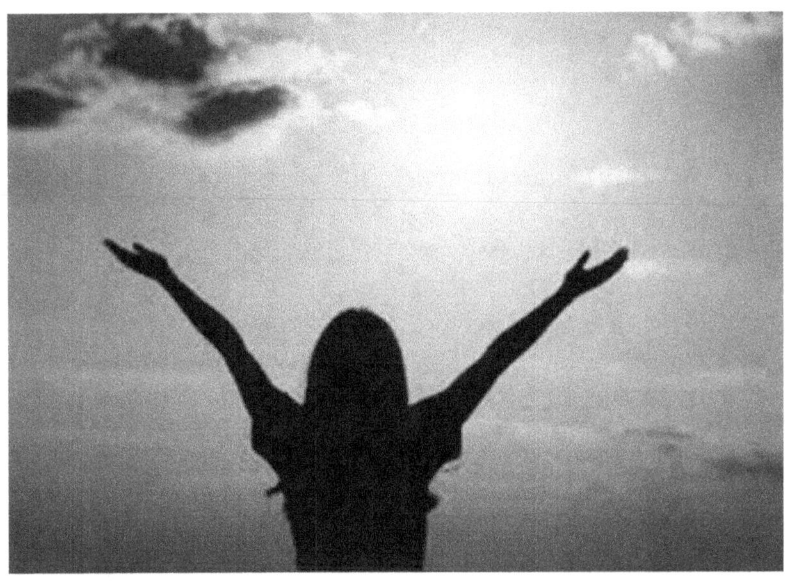

# MEDITATE AND REFLECT

## GOD IS LORD OF ALL

Matthew 6:24

No man can serve two masters: for either he will hate the one and love the other; or else he will hold to the one and despise the other. Ye cannot serve God and mammon.

## THOUGHT

As you grow in the grace of the Lord, your faith will be challenged. Where is your heart? Do you really believe in God and his promises for your life? We are not perfect, but we strive for perfection through Jesus Christ. It's amazing how we can come together to worship on a weekly basis but does the word of God really penetrate our hearts to where it can change situations around us? As believers, we walk by faith and not by sight. We come together as a body of believers to worship and bring God glory. We are created to love God with ALL our heart, mind, and soul. Through Christ, we have the power of God to pull down strongholds or anything that does not line up with the will

of the Lord.  Ultimately, God is the judge of us all and we must answer

to Him.

## PRAYER

Lord,

Teach us how to love you and live the life that you have purposed and ordained for us.  We are victorious and not just overcomers but more than conquerors.  There is nothing hidden in you.  We thank you for the precious blood that Jesus shed on Calvary that washes our sins.  We say thank you that we can come boldly before your throne and find mercy and grace.  Father teach us to love our enemy, despite of being misused.  We call on your name to save and deliver us.  In Jesus name.  Amen

# MY PERSONAL REFLECTIONS

## YOU ARE NOT REJECTED BUT ACCEPTED

PSALM 118:22

The stone which the builders refused is become the head stone of the

corner.

## THOUGHT

As we travel the journey of life, there will come a time where you may

feel left out, you may not belong or just rejected.  It is amazing that

God will never leave us.  However, we tend to leave the will of God.

God has called us to be separate, set apart and consecrated for HIS

purpose.  You may wonder why it appears that you may not "fit in" or

that you may not always go along with the "IN" crowd.  God has

stamped his approval on you!!!! You are sold out to do the will of God.

You are a light that shines in darkness.

## PRAYER

O God, let the light of your Holy Spirit burn bright within our hearts. Father, protect and shield us from hurt from our past and/or present of not being included (feeling accepted) or feeling of abandonment. We realize that we were created for purpose and destiny. Lord, place us firmly where you would want us to bring glory to your name. In Jesus name. Amen.

# MY PERSONAL REFLECTIONS

## YOU ARE VALUABLE

ISAIAH 40:29-31

29.  He giveth power to the faint; and to them that have no might he increaseth strength.

30.  Even the youth shall faint and be weary, and the young men shall utterly fall.

31.  But they that wait upon the LORD shall renew their strength: they shall mount up with wings as eagles; they shall run and not be weary and they shall walk and not faint.

## THOUGHT

God is our strength.  It's amazing that Abba Father God knows everything about you.  He knows even the number of hairs on your head.  God said that he would perfect that which concerneth you.  God is so AWESOME!  This is why we praise, sing and dance unto him.  God loves you so much!  When you are weak and downtrodden, God knows.  He is there to lift the burden and carry you.  No matter how big or small your circumstances, God will DELIVER YOU!

## PRAYER

Father God,

I love you and seek your face.  Thank you for hearing and answering my prayers.  Lord, I repent for all my sins and transgressions.  For I know, in your word that sin separates me from the love that you have for me.  Father, I ask that you cleanse me and make me whole for your name's sake.  Lord, I want to glorify you with my life.  I am a light that shines in darkness.  Lord allow me to glorify you in spirit and in truth so that my life would make a difference to someone.  In Jesus name. Amen.

# MY PERSONAL REFLECTIONS

**EVERYTHING MUST CHANGE**

ECCLESIATES 3:1

To everything there is a season and a time to every purpose under the heaven....

**THOUGHT**

As long as we have breath in our bodies, everything changes.  Nothing stays the same.  God Almighty has given us purpose with destiny to face changes that come into our lives.  Our focus as believers is to keep our minds on Jesus.  No matter what or whom we face, if we are living upright, God will see us through it.  We are predestined to fulfill the will of God in our lives.

**PRAYER**

Father,

In Jesus name, we seek your face for direction.  Thank you for hearing and answering our prayers.  Thank you, Lord, for the seasons that change, for it gives us a fresh outlook and perspective in life.  We know that tomorrow is not promised, and we thank you for every day and great expectations.  Lord, even though the seasons change we are glad that you do not change.  You are still great and mighty.  Thank you for caring so much for us and perfecting that concerns us.  In Jesus name. Amen.

## MY PERSONAL REFLECTIONS

# WHO DO YOU LOVE

~ 75 ~

JOHN 15:12-13

12.  This is my commandment, that ye love one another, as I have loved you.

13.   Greater love hath no man than this that a man lay down his life for his friends.

## THOUGHT

Have you fantasized of being in love with that special someone or ponder the idea of the meaning of true love?  What is the difference between love and lust?  Who do you openly give your heart to? Are you able to show love to the one who has mistreated you or lied to you or about you?  God has called us to love one another and walk in love. Who else would be a better example to follow than Jesus Christ?  He ultimately paid the price of love for us on Calvary.

**PRAYER**

Father,

Thank you for always hearing us when we pray to you.  Forgive us for everything that we have done that has separated us from the love that you have for us.  Forgive us for freely giving ourselves over to fornication, which we thought, was love but lust.  Renew our heart and teach us how to love you and to show that unconditional love to others. In Jesus name.  Amen.

# MY PERSONAL REFLECTIONS

## CAN WE GET ALONG

MATTHEW 5:11-12

11.  Blessed are you when people insult you, persecute you and falsely say all kinds of evil against you because of me.

12.  Rejoice and be glad, because great is your reward in heaven.

## THOUGHT

As you grow and mature in the Lord, your faith will be tested.  Whether you're being tested emotionally, physically, or spiritually; will you be able to stand?  Having done all, you can…STAND.  No matter what, hold your peace.  We know that we must let the fruits of the spirit operate in our lives. (Love, joy, peace, longsuffering, gentleness, goodness, faith, meekness, and temperance Galatians 5:22-23).  Do you know how to act and respond under pressure, insults or when that person has pressed that last nerve?  It is important that if we are going to be hearers of the word, we must be doers of the word as well.  God is watching our actions and reactions. Ultimately, Jesus is our foundation, and we must be rooted and grounded in him.

## PRAYER

Lord, we desire to hear from you and to know the leading of your calling. Thank you Lord, for shaping and molding us to do what you created us to do. As we grow in your word, there is a constant tearing down and building up of our minds and attitudes. Lord, please remove everything that is not like you. Cleanse and make us whole that we will be vessels of praise and honor for you. In Jesus name. Amen.

# MY PERSONAL REFLECTIONS

## TAKE A BREAK

EXODUS 33:13-14

13.  Shew me now thy way, that I may know thee.

14.  My presence shall go with thee, and I will give thee rest.

## THOUGHT

There are so many influences that overtake us day by day.  It may be friends, television shows, internet, cellular phones, and peer pressures to name a few.  All these things keep our minds so busy.  Stop!!! Take a break from everything to free your mind in the will of God.  Meditate on the things of God.  Seek God's face through prayer and studying the Holy Scriptures.  Let your mind be completely focused on God.  Allow yourself to rest in the presence of God and depend on his guidance.

**PRAYER**

Father, teach us that our expectancy is of you and not things or people in the world.  We want to rest and have peace and not bombarded with the busyness of everyday living.  We want to hear your voice.  Your voice will give us a calm spirit.  Let us rest in your presence.  In Jesus name.  Amen.

# MY PERSONAL REFLECTIONS

## WHERE ARE YOU GOING

EXODUS 33:13

Now therefore, I pray thee, if I have found grace in thy sight, shew me now thy way, that I may know thee, that I may find grace in thy sight: and consider that this nation is thy people.

ISAIAH 26:4

Trust ye in the LORD forever: for in the LORD JEHOVAH is everlasting strength.

MATTHEW 7:7-8

7. Ask and it shall be given you; seek and ye shall find; knock, and it shall be opened unto you:

8. For every one that asketh receiveth; and he that seeketh findeth; and to him that knocketh it shall be opened.

## THOUGHT

God is waiting ……ASK, SEEK, and KNOCK.  God longs for us to enter into his presence.  All that we will ever need; God has already provided.  The Lord has destined us for his purpose.  Your visions for the future are prepared for you to grasp hold.  It is important to learn and trust God in all aspects of life.  The journey of life lies ahead.  Allow God to lead you full speed ahead with prayer, fasting and strengthening yourself in The Word of God.

## PRAYER

Father, we come before you thanking you for who you are.  Lord, we desire to sup in your presence.  We humble ourselves before you so that you may pour into us.  Lord lead us on the path that you have predestined for our lives.  We put our hands in your hands.  Father lead us into the purpose and fulfillment of our destiny. We desire to give you the glory in all that we do and partake in. We call on your name. Hear our cries and have mercy for we desire to give you all the praise, honor, and glory. In the mighty name of Jesus. Amen.

# MY PERSONAL REFLECTIONS

# NOTES

# NOTES

Balch, P. (2010). *Prescriptions for nutritional healing.* (5th ed.). New York, NY: Penguin Group.

Ballentine, R. (2007). *Diet and nutrition.* Honesdale, PA: Himalayan Institute.

Bright, B. (2002). First *love.* Orlando, FL: New Life.

Cobb, B. (2002). *The living foods lifestyle.* Atlanta, GA: Living Soul.

*God's Principles of healthful living.* N.d. The restored church of God. Retrieved December 18, 2018

Lepore, D. (1985). *The ultimate healing system.* N. P Woodland.

Lipson, P. (2016, May 12). Naturopaths Fake Doctors In White Coats? *Forbes.*Retrieved

https:www.forbes.com/sites/peterlipson/2016/05/12/naturopaths-witch-Doctors-in-white-coats/#32ed663261

Omartian, S. (2002).*The power of a praying woman.* Eugene, OR: Harvest house.

Takahashi, T. (1989*). Atlas of the human body.* New York, NY: Woodland.

Thiel, R.  (2000). Naturopathy *for the 21st century*.  Warsaw, IN: Whitman.

White, E. G. (2007).  *The ministry of healing*.  Altamont, TN: Harvesttime.

Wright, H.  (2011). *A better way to think*.  Grand Rapids, MD: Revell.

# ABOUT THE AUTHOR

## Chiquilla Scott, N.D.

Chiquilla Scott is a Doctor of Naturopathy. She seeks to transform the world through natural health. She is the owner of Divine Virtue LLC where she specializes in natural health which provides holistic training to teach you to care for the body, mind, and spirit. She motivates, supports, and encourages others on their paths to healthier and happier lifestyles.

Natural health does not seek to diagnose, treat, cure, or prevent any disease, disorder or syndrome.

Dr. Chiquilla Scott operates Divine Virtue LLC as a natural and holistic Doctor of Naturopathy and Certified Health Coach. She specializes in providing natural health using natural, noninvasive techniques to promote wellbeing. The main focus is on natural health principles and techniques to support holistic wellness.

Common natural health techniques are nutrition, herbology, homeopathy and supplementation.

The doctor provides comprehensive health assessment, client education and nutritional consultation.

In her leisure time, she enjoys reading, writing, and running. She resides with her family in Atlanta, Georgia, which is also home of her alma mater, Clark Atlanta University.

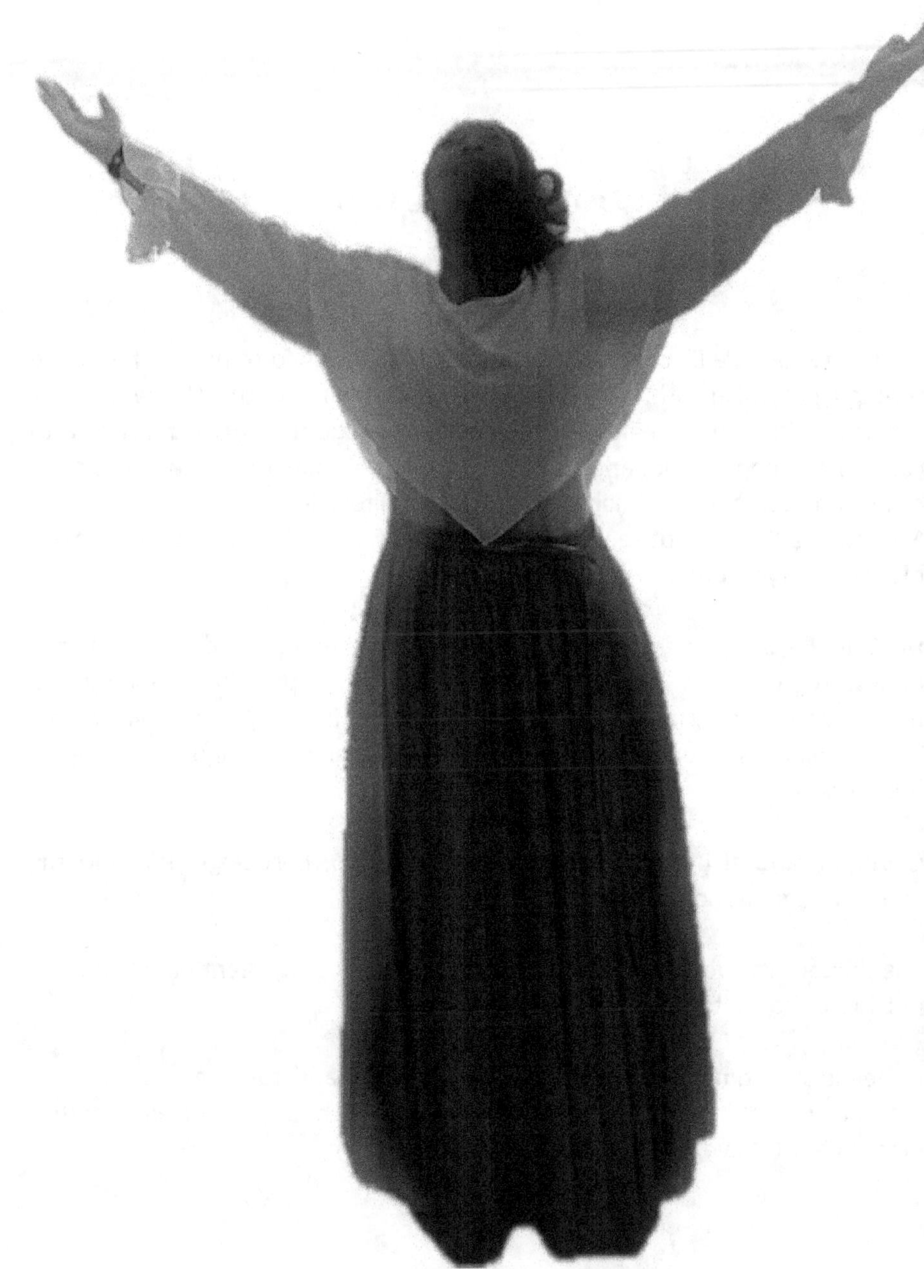

# NOTES

# NOTES

# NOTES

# NOTES

# NOTES